THE UGLY STORY
OF
CROHN's DISEASE

Gilles R. G. Monif, M.D.

TABLE of CONTENTS

TABLE of CONTENTS

PREFACE

In 2001, I stepped down as an Assistant Dean at Creighton University School of Medicine. Not ready to have the "little grey cells" undergo disuse atrophy, my research hobby, Infectious Diseases Incorporated, (IDI) and I ventured into the world of veterinary medicine where zoonotic infections make veterinary and human medicine kissing cousins.

IDI entered into a strategic partnership with the University of Florida College of Veterinary Medicine. The journey started with Johne's disease in cattle. Johne's disease is a chronic gastrointestinal disease due to *Mycobacterium avium* subspecies *paratuberculosis* (MAP) which was alleged to have crossed the zoonotic bridge between animals and humans and created disease in humans.

If the telling of Crohn's disease is somewhat laced with a touch of displeasure, it has to do with the lengths to which corporations will go to crush any threats to their bottom line. IDI joined with the Veterinary Research Institute (VRI) in the Czech Republic to pursue the issues embedded in MAP and Crohn's disease. VRI's infectious disease section was led by an internationally acknowledged thought leader, Professor Karel Hruska. The VRI group had published the key that that stood to unlock the mechanism of spread underlying the Crohn's disease epidemic. They identified that 49% of 51 brands of infant formula manufactured by 10 producers in seven different countries contained MAP. In December of 2012, overnight the directors and department chairs within the Veterinary Research Institute's section dealing with zoonotic mycobacterial diseases and *Mycobacterium avium* subspecies *paratuberculosis* were suspended without any stated reason being given. Its internationally respected director, Professor Karel Hruska, was pressured into premature retirement. Professor Hruska would later write *"Details are not needed; nobody would believe them. It is an absurd theatre"*.

The other professional assassinations were subtle: loss of grant support, a visit by a university president, the loss of employment, etc. The "VRI massacre" was a blatant bludgeoning of science that should not be allowed to quietly pass into the night. Disruption of a

1

committed collaboration between Veterinary Research Institute (VRI) of the Czech Republic and Infectious Diseases Incorporated (IDI) of the United States left IDI the last voice standing. I had to have long discussions with all my children and wife with regard to the risks of going forward. I entered medicine when it was in its golden age. Now medicine's moral compass vacillates between tarnished copper and something resembling rusting iron., What happened in the Czech Republic underscored the need to get into print as much information about Crohn's disease as possible.

Crohn's disease was once the poster-boy of autoimmunity. We now know that it is not true. The mechanism by which MAP induces an immune-mediated disease stands to potentially liberate other alleged "autoimmune diseases" (rheumatoid arthritis, psoriasis, thyroiditis, etc.) from the paralysis imposed by their being so labeled.

The complexity of the factors involved in telling the story of Crohn's disease threatens to challenge the reader. The individual components of the Crohn's disease enigma are presented as a mosaic of information. They come together to tell why Crohn's disease is the disease that should have never been.

The book is dedicated to Karel Hruska, Ivo Pavlik, Ron Chiodini, John Hermon-Taylor, and Saleh Naser who chose not to sin by silence.

CROHN'S DISEASE

Dr Burrill Bernard Crohn and his two colleagues, Dr Gordon Oppenheimer and Dr Leon Ginzburg have been formally credited with the discovery of the disease (1932). The disease takes its name from Dr Burrill B Crohn.

Crohn's disease is one of two inflammatory-type diseases of the intestines cared for primarily by gastroenterologists.

Factual Introduction to Crohn's Disease

- Prior to the 1930s, Crohn's disease was so rare that it basically escaped medical detection.
- Crohn's disease is an inflammatory bowel disease of the human gastrointestinal tract. It primarily affects the ileocecal portion of the small bowel, and less frequently, the first portion of the large bowel.
- One in every four afflicted individuals will have one or more operations to remove diseased bowel.
- The characteristic age of onset is between 11-24 years of age. A second, smaller group presents at a time of waning immunity late in life. Currently, an earlier age of onset is being identified in children.
- Crohn's disease is a lifelong affliction.
- Like most diseases, the genetic governance of inherent immunity defines individual susceptibility.
- Crohn's disease is now a global epidemic within industrialized nations. In 2002, the CDC estimated the number of US cases of Crohn's disease at 200,000. A decade later the number of active cases surpassed 800,000. Today there are over 1.2 million cases in the United States and that number increases annually.
- Crohn's disease is rare in third world economies until the introduction of western diets.
- The number of new cases of Crohn's disease is increasing worldwide.
- In the United States, the medical costs of Crohn's disease have been reported to be $12,000 - $18,000 a year.

- In the United States, the annual medical and indirect costs had once been estimated at $15 billion and $4.2 billion respectively.
- The cost of care for individuals afflicted with Crohn's disease (not covered by insurance) is being assumed by the federal government, and indirectly, by the tax payers.
- Because of its socioeconomic and public health importance, Johne's disease had been listed by the Office International des Epizooties (OIE) as a category B pathogen.

What fact sheets do not say is that Crohn's disease is a destroyer of lives and sometimes life itself. Living becomes knowing where every toilet exists. Careers are sacrificed to accommodate the disease. Individuals are often obliged to leave the workforce in their prime earning years. One person's story marked me. He developed Crohn's disease at age 11. He was put on prolonged courses of steroids. Steroids are a two-edged knife. Misused, the consequences can be tragic. Prolonged courses of steroids caused physical and mental changes that destroyed much of his sense of self-worth. He prematurely terminated his life. As a physician, not knowing what you are doing therapeutically can transform the attempt to do good into something totally unintended.

THE QUEST FOR CAUSATION

The United States contribution to the story of Crohn's disease began in 1989. Ron Chiodini published a paper in which he noted the similarity of a gastrointestinal disease in cattle (Johne's disease) due to Crohn's disease. Because of its socioeconomic and public health importance, Johne's disease had long been listed by the **Office International des Epizooties (OIE)** as a **category B pathogen.**

Exploring the possibility that MAP might be the cause of Crohn's disease, Chiodini and Rossiter in 1996 successfully isolated MAP from the feces of 26 out of 135 patients with Crohn's disease, but from only one of 121 control individuals. These findings became the underpinnings of the U.S. infectious disease paradigms of causation for Crohn's disease. Greater credibility to this postulate was added in 2000 when Naser and co-investigators isolated MAP only from the breastmilk of women with Crohn's disease.

The idea that an animal mycobacterium could become a human pathogen had previously been documented. In the early 1900s, a bovine mycobacterium, **Mycobacterium bovis**, became a significant threat to the public welfare. *M. bovis* bridged the gap between domestic animals and humans through it being shed into the milk produced by infected animals. Between 1912 and 1937, an estimated 65,000 individuals in England and Wales died from gastrointestinal disease contracted from the consumption of milk containing *M. bovis*. Corresponding figures for the United States are not available, but one is engraved in the bedrock of my personal memory.

The initial response to this threat to the public welfare was initially addressed by instituting a policy of testing animals *for M. bovis*. If an animal was found to be infected, the entire herd was destroyed. The threat created for the public welfare and milk-based agribusiness was resolved when it was demonstrated that *M. bovis* could be destroyed by pasteurization.

In the late 1980s, multiple studies documented that, not only could an infected animal shed MAP into its milk, but the MAP in milk was not effectively destroyed by pasteurization. The rate of culture recovery of

MAP from raw and pasteurized milk was demonstrated to be virtually identical. The Marshfield Clinic Retail Milk Study is reputed to have demonstrated viable MAP in 2.8% of milk samples taken directly from grocery stores in three of the nation's largest dairy states.

The demonstration of viable MAP in milk constituted a real and eminent threat to the dairy industry and, more significantly, to the manufacturers of dairy protein-based products. The industrialization of milk production had rendered the re-introduction of the United Kingdom's methodology of test-and-cull and herd eradication economically unfeasible. Pressure is alleged to have been brought to silence the issue. Ron Choidini lost his grant support. He ultimately left investigative research for over a decade.

In 1997, a group of USDA scientists, headed by Judith Stabel, published a paper claiming that high temperature/short duration pasteurization used in the United States destroyed MAP. The methodology used was quickly criticized for having been designed to attain a predictable outcome. The USDA scientists had taken frozen, not fresh, MAP organisms and then sonicated them prior to adulterating the milk samples to be tested.

The United Kingdom's story of Crohn's disease has its foundation with John Hermon-Taylor's publication of a case of MAP lymph adenitis in a boy who five years later developed a terminal ileitis. Two years later, his publications had the titles which delineated his perception of causation: *Causation of Crohn's disease by Mycobacterium avium subspecies paratuberculosis, Mycobacterium avium subspecies paratuberculosis is the causation of Crohn's disease,* and *Mycobacterium avium subspecies paratuberculosis is a cause of Crohn's disease.*

The reputation of John Hermon-Taylor was a factor in focusing the United Kingdom's perspective on whether MAP constituted a public health hazard. Referring to Crohn's disease, Lord Justice Phillip's 2001 report to Her Majesty's government stated *"Where the likelihood of a risk to human life may appear remote, where there is uncertainty, all reasonably precautionary measures should not be played down on the grounds that the risk is unproven".* Similar concerns were stated in the United Kingdom Food Standards Agency report: *"There is undoubtedly sufficient cause for concern* (referring to MAP and Crohn's disease) *for further action to be urgently taken to determine what the available data means.... This question can be divided into two areas: What actions should be taken to reduce exposure to MAP even though the causal link is not established; and what actions can be taken to increase the knowledge base so that future decisions may be made upon more information".*

In late 2000 and early 2001, the United States Congress held hearings to determine whether MAP constituted a potential hazard to the public health. In step with the United Kingdom, Congress determined that sufficient evidence existed to warrant substantial funding (ultimately an estimated 90 million dollars) to *"increase the knowledge base so that future decisions may be made upon more information".*

The discredited USDA publication, contending that the way milk is pasteurized in the U.S. was safe, resurfaced in congressional hearings. It became part of an extensive lobbying campaign that redirected funding from the National Institutes of Health to USDA. USDA was given sole stewardship to determine whether a bovine pathogen that had penetrated the nation's food supply constituted a risk to the public welfare.

BELLEVUE HOSPITAL

The first piece of the Crohn's disease mosaic occurred during my rotation in pathology during my first-year internship on the Columbia Internal Medicine Service at Bellevue Hospital in New York City.

The resident I had been assigned to work with failed to show up. I had seen him on a Tuesday. Wednesday, he missed the appointment. He had what was then called idiopathic enterocolitis or regional enteritis. At twenty-five, David had already had surgery to remove diseased bowel. That surgery resulted in his small bowel being so repositioned that when his disease penetrated the intestinal wall, its contents spilled into the peritoneal cavity and not the cul-de-sac. He died due to overwhelming sepsis. In 1961, his disease was called regional enteritis or iatrogenic enterocolitis. These diagnoses reflected a collection of letters behind which resided the then collective medical ignorance. Today his disease is known as Crohn's disease.

The next piece of the mosaic was Lucy Garcia. She was twenty-two years old, about five feet five inches tall with long jet-black hair and big oval brown eyes. She made a beautiful canvas, blemished only by her swollen ankles. The curved elegance of well-turned ankles was absent. In their place were pipe-like enlargements that fused into her calves. By mental exclusion based on the physical examination and urine analysis, the only site that had the surface area to affect a massive loss of blood protein was the gastrointestinal tract. The inflammatory disease entity that fit was regional enteritis. A bribe to the night radiology technician got me the films that showed massive involvement of the ileocecal area. The next day , the attending physician had but to agree. The Gastrointestinal Service put a protein called albumin with a radio-labeled tag into her blood stream. Large amounts of the tag were identified in her feces.

Regional enteritis was then one of those diseases about which we did not understand the hows and whys, but treated to the best of our knowledge. In 1961, the terms idiopathic or regional enteritis were used to hide the fact that we had no idea what were the events that combined to produce disease. Lucy was given the then wonder drugs

9

of the 1960s, corticosteroids. Shortly thereafter, I was rotated to the male ward. Five weeks later, I got a call from the senior administrative resident for the female ward.

"Do you remember Lucy Garcia?

A little hesitant, I asked , "Why".

"She died! She had regional enteritis, all right, but it was due to the type of tuberculosis you get from drinking unpasteurized milk (*Mycobacterium bovis*). There was no PPD (a skin test for tuberculosis due to *Mycobacterium tuberculosis*) in the chart!

"I thought you would want to know!"

The steroids were the firing squad. The responsibility for her being there was mine. Her death sensitized me to diseases caused by mycobacteria. Even though years later I perceived that a PPD to tuberculosis had but weak cross-reactivity with *Mycobacterium bovis,* that guilt etched *a* permanent place in my memory.

Years later, that administrative resident would become Vice President and Dean at Creighton University School of Medicine and I a Professor of Obstetrics and Gynecology.

Little did I realize that Lucy would be my introduction to the world of zoonosis. **Zoonosis** refers to **zoonotic** diseases that can be passed from animals to humans. Animals can carry harmful germs, such as bacteria, fungi, parasites, and viruses. These are then shared with humans and cause illness and possible death. *Mycobacterium* bovis is a zoonotic pathogen. Infection/disease is most frequently acquired by oral ingestion of the organism resulting in gastrointestinal disease as its primary clinical manifestation. In the Middle Ages, the fashion of very high collars covering the entire neck was due to tuberculous mycobacterial infection of the regional lymph nodes causing disfiguring masses and fistulae (scrofula).

THE NATIONAL INSTITUTES OF HEALTH

In 1963, the Berlin Wall and direct confrontation with Russia was in play. Being one of the youngest residents at Bellevue Hospital in New York City, being drafted was a certainty. How and why would become part of the next mosaic piece.

The garage for Bellevue Hospital faces First Avenue: six lanes of on-coming traffic. To cross First Avenue and make two immediate left to get downtown using Second Avenue requires white knuckle driving. One evening on leaving Bellevue Hospital, I caught out of the corner of my eye that someone had just pulled the same maneuver as I had. When I turned left onto Second Avenue, the other vehicle did the same. After enough lane changes and turns, the word coincidence was no longer valid. Later, the extra click of my parent's telephone telegraphed a different meaning. Once my top security cleared, I was informed that I was being drafted for the U.S. Army's Biological Warfare Laboratories at Camp Detrick (In the 1960s, the Vellum 1B strain of anthrax was being developed as a bioweapon for the UK and the US). Thank you, but no-thank you, rerouted me to the National Institutes of Health in Bethesda, Maryland.

I was assigned to the laboratory of Dr, John Severs. That was an incredible landing spot. A means of identifying rubella virus had just been identified and the world was in the midst of a congenital rubella epidemic. Three different groups (Walter Reed, Harvard, and NICHD) were locked in a battle of egos.

Part of my benchwork training involved becoming proficient with all the culture and serological tools applicable to medical virology. One diagnostic technique captured my interest. For the identification of the Coxsackie viruses, one-day old suckling mice needed to be used. If a Coxsackie virus was present in the challenge material injected into its abdomen, the baby mouse would die. But if I injected a two-day-old suckling mouse with the same amount of virus or even three times the amount, nothing happened. "WHY" intrigued me.

In the 1950s and 1960s, rubella virus was the global panic disease entity. In children and adults, rubella is no big deal: short term, a low-grade temperature, occasional aching joints associated with a characteristic rash. These signs and symptoms quickly disappear leaving no untoward consequences. If a woman contracted rubella early in her pregnancy and the virus crossed the placental barrier and infected the fetus, the devastating consequences were collectively termed the congenital rubella syndrome. What occurred to suckling mice was the product of experimentation. Congenital rubella syndrome was an experiment in nature in which there was no possibility of investigator manipulation. What infants with congenital rubella and suckling mice shared in common was the absence of acquired immunity.

My military service produced a dozen peer-reviewed publications describing the pathogenesis of congenital rubella and the first book ever published on viral infections of the human fetus (*Viral Infections of the Human Fetus*).

THE UNIVERSITY OF FLORIDA COLLEGE OF MEDICINE

My rotation through pathology convinced me that the great diagnosticians in medicine were not internists but pathologists i.e. William Osler and Marvin Kuskner. Being already known to the Department of Pathology at New York University School of Medicine, I was accepted to do a pathology residency.

My past at the NIH followed me. During my residency, the Chairman of the Department of Obstetrics and Gynecology, Harry Prystowski, engaged in an aggressive a two-year campaign to recruit me (Dr. Prystowski ultimately became Vice President of the University of Pennsylvania). Trying to get him to stop calling, I gave him a set of requirements that I was certain would never be met. Wrong! Trained as an internist, pathologist and immunologist, instead of becoming an Assistant Professor of Pathology or a chief resident, I became an Assistant Professor of Obstetrics and Gynecology at the University of Florida College of Medicine. The conditions of my employment were such that I owed Dr. Prystowski one hour per week. My charge was to bring infectious disease discipline to obstetrics and gynecology.

The bacterial flora of the female genital tract was characterized and quantitated. Protocols for the prophylactic use of antibiotics, treatment of endomyometritis, antibiotic selection etc. were developed and implemented. In 1975, the medical text book, *Infectious Diseases in Obstetrics and Gynecology* (currently in its sixth edition) won the medical writers award for best multi-authored medical text. The Infectious Disease Society for Obstetrics and Gynecology and its international counterpart were co-founded. Service was rendered to the American College of Obstetricians and Gynecologists as its special interest consultant on infectious disease as well as occasional consultant to the CDC.

Three things came out of the University of Florida experience that would have significance in solving the Crohn's disease enigma.

Delivery of a baby through a birth canal harboring either of the *Herpes simplex* viruses had the potential to induce a systemic infection in the baby that often culminated in death. With Marvin Amstey, guidelines were developed to preclude such an event from happening. The analysis of neonatal morbidity and mortality established that **human acquired immunity becomes functional around the fourth week of life**.

The second contribution came from the demonstration of how a change in **the microbiological environment could weaponize constituents of what is otherwise a symbiotic bacterial flora**. Infectious disease specialists in internal medicine had long treated men and women with acute gonococcal infection the same. They failed to take into account the anatomical and microbiological differences in play. The male urethra is a sterile, aerobic microbiological environment. Only when inflammation is advanced are aerobic skin organisms recruited into the process resulting in healing by fibrosis. The female genital tract is a much more elongated glandular conduit beginning at the endocervix and ending with the open terminal ends of the fallopian tubes. The endocervix has intimate contact with the vaginal flora of the female genital tract. What was demonstrated was that the changes in the local microbiological environment induced by the gonococcus serially weaponized constituents within the bacterial flora of the female genital tract. The resultant tissue damage could result in ectopic pregnancy, secondary infertility or tubo-ovarian abscesses. The female endocervix has access to the female genital tract flora. The decision was made not to base therapy exclusively on the microbiological data which was at the front of the conduit, but rather by encompassing the potential pathogenic spectrum of the anaerobic progression. The CDC's radical revamping of its therapeutic recommendation for pelvic inflammatory disease was written collaboratively on my dining room table in Gainesville Florida. By therapeutically encompassing the various bacterial species that function within the anaerobic progression, much morbidity and mortality due to sexually transmitted diseases have been circumvented.

The third contribution came in the form of a friendship with **Joseph Elliot Williams**. The friendship began one cold, windy January day at a bass fishing tournament. When the pairing was completed, two individuals were left. Neither had a boat. I had an electric trolling motor at my cabin at Cross Creek. We rented a boat. We would alternate. One person fished while the another held the electric trolling motor from falling into Orange Lake. Elliot won the tournament and I came in a respectable fifth. Elliot was a laboratory technician at the University of Florida College of Veterinary Medicine. Had he not been a military brat, had to move every two to four years and had the education opportunities open to most, I would be referring to him as Professor Williams. Elliot too was a Trekkie who liked to go where no one had gone before. He would later be my passport into the world of veterinary medicine and *Mycobacterium avium* subspecies *paratuberculosis*.

MYCOBACTERIUM AVIUM SUBSPECIES PARATUBERCULOSIS

Mycobacterium avium subspecies *paratuberculosis* (MAP) belongs to the group of mycobacteria that are theorized to have evolved from *Mycobacterium avium*. The microbe's reservoir is in soil and contaminated water. Not surprisingly, MAP infection has been identified in almost every herbivore studied in depth: cows, sheep, goats, deer elk, buffalo, camels, etc. Grass-feeding animals, both wild and domestic, ingesting the organism, become infected. When certain conditions are met, a small number of infected animals develop a chronic granulomatous infection of their gastrointestinal tract. The gastrointestinal tract of animals, as well as humans, contains complementary receptor sites that allow MAP to attach to the gastrointestinal mucosa.

In domestic animals, the disease due to MAP is called Johne's disease. Johne's disease is a chronic inflammatory disease of the gastrointestinal tract. Diseased animals develop soft stools that eventually progress to profuse diarrhea. If allowed to run its course, the disease is usually terminal. *Mycobacterium avium* subspecies *paratuberculosis* (MAP) infection of domestic animals has long been a major veterinary challenge. Bovine MAP infection results in lower cow fertility, lower calf weight, and lower weaning calf weight. MAP infection results in incremental declines in reproduction, milk production, and fat content. Once subclinical MAP infection becomes clinically overt (**Johne's disease**), the animal's life expectancy is numbered in terms of weeks. Often, diseased animals are shipped to slaughter houses just prior to their demise. In 1999, MAP's cost to milk producers was an estimated 1.5 billion dollars. Almost two decades later, the widespread prevalence of MAP within milk-producing herds substantially increased the so-called "MAP Milk Tax".

The demonstrated universal presence of these receptor sites within the gastrointestinal tract has explained the ease with which MAP can cross species barriers. Human MAP isolates, having been demonstrated to have similar genetic markers to animal MAP isolates, made it, more probable than not, that MAP isolates cultured from human beings could produce disease in susceptible animals and vice versa.

Johne's disease was front and center a priority concern of the global veterinary community. Because of the socioeconomic and public health importance, The Office International des Epizooties (OIE) had listed paratuberculosis (the disease caused by MAP) as a disease of major global importance. Veterinarians and allied scientists had banded together in forming the **International Paratuberculosis Association** Paratuberculosis was categorized as a List B pathogen in terms of its socioeconomic and/or public health importance.

ENTRY INTO THE WORLD
OF VETERINARY MEDICINE

Distance had never been a barrier. Elliot and I kept in contact on both a personal and professional level. He began working for a distinguished, veterinary pathologist at the University of Florida College of Veterinary Medicine, Claus D. Buergelt. His research centered on *Mycobacterium avium* subspecies *paratuberculosis*(MAP). By virtue of his employment, Claus's interests became Elliot's. Elliot's frustration with the status quo became mine. When not focused on fishing, our correspondence often involved Elliot's work. In retrospect, he was slowly playing out the bait to me.

Initially, I was a little south of ignorant when it came to MAP. When you are not interested in a subject, you tend to be a slow learner or "capta dura" (thick headed). Exchanges about MAP did not graciously transcend the barriers of time and distance. When they did, I got it. MAP had the potential to be an incredible two-headed dragon: one, a threat to the national economy and the second, a threat to the public health. What I could accomplish for the discipline of Obstetrics and Gynecology had run its course. Having kept a house in the fishing community of Cedar Key made returning to Florida sort of a homecoming. Using prior relationships at the University of Florida, in 2001, IDI entered into a strategic partnership with the university to study MAP. Charles Courtney, Associate Dean for Research, gave me a courtesy faculty appointment in the Department of Pathobiology of the College of Veterinary Medicine as a Visiting Scientist.

The Laboratory of Professor Claus Buergelt controlled The Veterinary Diagnostic Laboratory for Paratuberculosis at the University of Florida College of Veterinary Medicine. Coincidence had it that Claus was also the treasurer of the **International Paratuberculosis Association**.

The initial passport into Dr. Buergelt's laboratory was Elliot's strong recommendation. Claus was initially a bit reserved about the IDI invasion. He was true to his German heritage, He was a strong believer in the law of gravity: nothing was supposed to defy that law, including innovative ideas. Claus's fear of being in error had frustrated Elliot and compromised the laboratories funding. Seed money for MAP and Crohn's disease came from IDI.

Despite our divergent French and German heritages, Claus and I developed a relationship of mutual respect. Claus would later describe me to other faculty members as the scientist from Mars.

The MAP diagnostic area was a mess. You could have an animal with Johne's disease and negative serological test or an animal with a positive diagnostic serological and no evidence of MAP. The alleged pathogenesis of Johne's disease was envisioned as a three- stage progress from infection to disease occurring over many months or years. The proposed natural history of MAP was different from that of other pathogenic mycobacteria. Only Mycobacteria leprae had any overlapping features. What eventually was documented that USDA had certified diagnostic tests that identified primarily animals with but a reasonable probability of developing Johne's disease. USDA's insistence that only mycobacteria with the IS900 insertion sequence could cause Johne's disease resulted in the non-detection of genomic variants that did. USDA facilitated the widespread dissemination of MAP into previously uninfected herds by embracing technology that had effectively masked the presence and prevalence of MAP. Not requiring a statement as to whether an animal was infected by MAP on its heath certificate allowed infected animals to be shipped across state and even national borders. The Japanese Health officials have documented that 54% of MAP infected cows imported to Japan came from the United States. Once new diagnostic technology was in place, it could be documented that the natural history of MAP was comparable to that of tuberculosis in which many are infected but few develop disease.

Academically, the IDI/FU collaboration produced over thirty peer and non-peer review academic publications and four U.S patents. But more important, it provided the background pieces that filled in gaps for the construction of the Hruska Postulate.

USDA

A way of dealing with an uncomfortable problem is to create a committee to study it with the hope that in the ensuing interim the problem will either solve itself or be forgotten. UDSA proceeded to institute a volunteer test-and-cull program. In April of 2002, USDA-APHIS implemented the Uniform Program Standards for the Volunteer Bovine Johne's Disease Control Program and instituted a five-year Johne's Disease Prevention Dairy Herd Demonstration Program. In addressing MAP's potential threat to agribusiness, USDA made a number of administrative decisions that have inflicted substantial long-term damage to the nation's milk producing herds.

- In 2000, almost 20% of the milk-producing dairy herds in the United States contained MAP infected animals. USDA did two things to assure that number would not be static. First, USDA certified MAP diagnostic tests that, under the best of circumstances, identified only 30% of infected animals. Secondly, USDA refused to require that an animal's MAP status be a requisite on its health certificate. Quality of merchandise issues for livestock is addressed through the process of health certification of the animal. Revisions to part 71 and 80 of the Code of Federal Registration restrict interstate movement of MAP infected animals except to recognized slaughter establishments. Not testing an animal prevented an impediment to interstate transportation of an infected animal. With respect to MAP, an animal's certificate of health needed the words "buyer beware" to be added. Contrary to the Animal Health Protection Act (7 U.S.C. 8301 et seq.), USDA's decision permitted infected animals to be transported across national borders with relative ease and introduced into non-infected milking herds.
- In 2002, USDA estimated that between 20-30% of U.S. dairy herds contained MAP infected animals.
- In 2007, the National Health Monitoring System of 515 dairy farms demonstrated that 31.2% of participating dairy farms had bulk tank milk that tested positive for MAP.

- In 2007, USDA acknowledged that an estimated 70% of U.S. dairy herds contained MAP infected animals.
- In 2008, USDA introduced the National Johne's Disease Control Program whose three goals were 1) Reduce the prevalence of MAP /Johne's disease, 2) Reduce the impact of Johne's disease on individual herds and 3) Reduce introducing Johne's disease to uninfected herds. This program became referred to as "The Cow/MAP is out of the Barn/Why Now Lock the Door Program."
- In 2012, 54% of the animals identified in quarantine as being MAP infected had been exported to Japan from the United States
- In 2012, OIE contemplated removing paratuberculosis from the Terrestrial Animal Health Code because *"MAP infection is so widespread, continued recognition of MAP as an animal pathogen would only cause economic losses through the restriction in international trade".*
- By 2015, the number of large U.S. herds containing MAP-infected animals was estimated to exceed 90%.
- In 2018, more likely than not,it approaches 100%

Despite a growing body of evidence, the veterinary response to MAP as a possible hazard to the public welfare had a muted voice. Even if the topic was ever mentioned, it came with the CYA phrase "lack of conclusive proof ".

From 2001 to 2018, USDA took a once manageable problem and made it into one of colossal proportions. Today, no large dairy operation in the United States is MAP free and the number of infected animals within a given herd is significant. Its policies being neither economically feasible nor capable of eliminating MAP from milking herds, USDA rested on its laurels. An expensive $90,000,000 fact gathering program lost its reason for being, but not without creating consequences.

Viewed from a different perspective, the group at Ames in charge of decision making for MAP and Johne's disease held true to the agency's mission: to advance and protect agribusiness Whether it be with anthrax, bovine tuberculosis, toxigenic E. coli, etc., whenever USDA intervenes, it does so because the infectious disease process in question constitutes a threat to agribusiness. The real USDA is composed of hardworking men and women who are dedicated to their craft. IDI could not have accomplished as much as it did with the local USDA support. Literally under the table, the Florida USDA veterinarians gave IDI access to serum and fecal samples from the Florida Johne's Disease Prevention Dairy Herd Demonstration Program.

USDA's certified diagnostic tests lacked sensitivity for the detection of MAP. IDI obtained serum samples from a herd that had been enrolled for four years in USDA's Florida Dairy Demonstration Project and certified as being MAP/Johne's disease free. The State of Florida Veterinary Diagnostic Center confirmed the MAP-free status of the first herd using the best of the two U.S. certified diagnostic tests. The Veterinary Diagnostic Laboratory of the University of Florida College of Veterinary Medicine (UFCVM) used by IDI identified 10 animals as having had or having MAP infection.

USDA gave official certification to tests whose high positive results correlated , at very best, with a reasonable probability of that animal progressing to disease. Neither USDA nor the test manufacturers ever answered the question as to the significance of a negative test result. The IDI/USDA data subsequently demonstrated that the majority of infected animals ceased to have evidence of active infection. Only a small number of infected animals continued to have serological evidence of active infection. The period of study was too short to identify how many of these animals would have developed Johne's disease.

Using an IDI newly developed serum test that distinguished passive from active infection, IDI was able to determine that the Whitlock/Buergelt natural history of Johne's disease was in error. MAP's natural history was comparable to that described for tuberculosis (*Mycobacterium tuberculosis*). *Disease was but the top of an iceberg. When overt disease was present, it occurred in herds that already had a significant number of sub-clinically infected animals. Even though the study design and data integration were done by IDI, the right to publication resided with USDA. The USDA/Ames never chose to publish the data.*

Equally disconcerting was the occasional absence of MAP antibodies in animals with tissue-documented Johne's disease. USDA/Ames had made the internal decision that MAP was The and Only cause of Johne's disease. Other mycobacteria derived from the Mycobacterium avium evolutionary tree were but environmental contaminants. In building its ELISA blood test to detect the presence of MAP antibodies and its nested PCR tests for the detection of antigen, IDI expanded the antigen spectrum of its test to cover *M. hominissuis* and *Mycobacterium avium*. When tested in USDA's Laboratory Certification Testing , the blood test had a 100% correlation. The PCR test results were such that the University Florida Veterinary Diagnostic Laboratory using IDI's PCR tests was one of only two laboratories to be certified.

Despite documented superiority, IDI's tests did not come to market because the cost of going against the established MAP diagnostic tests was projected to be overly expensive given the established competition, the limited market and test manufacturers' close association with Ames. In a USDA semi-closed session held in conjunction with the 10th International Colloquium on Paratuberculosis (Johne's disease), the maker of the dominate MAP ELISA test requested that USDA allow their test to become the reference gold standard against which all MAP testing would be evaluated.

THE INFECTIOUS DISEASE POSTULATE OF CAUSATION

The veterinary world provided a key piece of information. MAP must become prevalent within the milk-producing herds before Crohn's disease appears in the general population. Iceland is the best epidemiologic demonstration of this point Prior to the German "co-habitation" of Iceland, the disease caused by MAP in domestic animals had been undetected. In 1933, the Germans brought sheep to Iceland, some of which were infected by this organism. With time, MAP disease became epidemic in sheep and eventually in cattle. The incidence of Crohn's disease in Iceland from 1950-1959 was 0.4 cases per 100,000 individuals per year; from 1960-1969 0.9; from 1970-1979 3.1; from 1980-1989 3.11 and from 1990-1995 5.6.

From 2000-2008, the medical infectious disease postulate of causation of Crohn's disease gained significant credibility. In 2002, Naser recovered isolated MAP from the breastmilk of two women with Crohn's disease, but not from controls. Three years later, Naser et al. (co-workers) cultured MAP from the blood of 50% of patients with Crohn's disease, 22% of individuals with ulcerative colitis and 0% of individuals without inflammatory bowel disease. In a subsequent follow up study done in conjunction with two other testing facilities (one being that of the Center for Disease Control and Prevention), MAP was identified in the blood of 22 out of 40 individuals with inflammatory bowel disease, **but also from 4 of 18 subjects with other problems.** Sechi et al., Bull et al. Autschack et al. identified a positive correlation between demonstration of MAP in diseased tissue and Crohn's disease. But, MAP DNA was identified in gastrointestinal tissue derived from a small number of individuals who did not have Crohn's disease. Scana et al. presented circumstantial evidence incriminating MAP in the pathogenesis of "irritable bowel disease".

In 2008, the American Academy of Microbiologists published its report, ***Mycobacterium avium paratuberculosis: Infrequent Human Pathogen or Public Health Threat***. Its executive summary states "*the association of MAP and CD is no longer in question. The critical issue is* *not whether MAP is associated with CD, but whether MAP causes CD or is incidentally present".*

The demonstration of MAP DNA within diseased gastrointestinal tissue from Crohn's afflicted individuals was but inferential. The detection of MAP within non-disease gastrointestinal tissue from either healthy individuals or individuals with other diseases was damning. **A "medical truth" (error-to-date) must account for the exceptions as well as those sustaining the hypothesis.** The presence of MAP in gastrointestinal tissues from individuals without clinical Crohn's disease required answers.

The death blow to the **direct MAP infectious disease paradigm came from the inability, using standard culture technology, to isolate or identify, using special stains, MAP organism in diseased gastrointestinal** tissue from individuals with Crohn's disease. In Johne's disease, MAP is readily cultured and demonstrable in diseased gastrointestinal tissue from animals with Johne's disease; same organism, different mechanisms causing disease.

THE PHARMACEUTICAL INDUSTRY

The pharmaceutical industry is a hot-bed of creativity and innovation. It is a sharp two-edged sword.

My introduction to the pharmaceutical industry came while I was an Assistant Professor at the University of Florida. Pfizer had developed a tetracycline, doxycycline, to compete with aureomycin® In studying the antibiotic susceptibility of constituents of the anaerobic progression, I identified that doxycycline had significant anerobic coverage and a renal mode of excretion that fit into the developing schema for sexually transmitted diseases of women. I shared this information with Pfizer and outlined for them how to market the drug. The rest is history. Today, doxycycline is firmly entrenched in the world's antibiotic arsenal. Pfizer could not do enough for me. It was a near perfect marriage. Pfizer used me for product promotion and I used Pfizer to disseminate information relative to the proper therapy for women with sexually transmitted diseases. Pfizer published and distributed free some 30,000 copies of the resident handbook on infectious diseases in obstetrics and gynecology throughout a number of countries.

Years later when I decided to leave the University of Florida, I was offered medical directorship of Pfizer's European operations. The temptation was great: a French heritage, a French wife, and the opportunity for my children to receive a European education. But by then, the pharmaceutical industry had moved beyond just pushing the envelope on indications or creating a de novo market. The age of antibiotics which produced ampicillin carbenicillin clindamycin , metronidazole, aminoglycosides, etc. and antimicrobials had lost its fiscal luster and profitability by curing diseases. The industry became focused on chronic disease and drugs that palliated, but did not cure. Chronic diseases are cash cows. Curing kills profitability. Outside of vaccines, there is little to no profit in prevention.

Even in the area of vaccines, therapeutic objectives had changed. The rubella and polio virus vaccines had documented that RNA live-vaccines conferred life-long immunity. For RNA viruses, the emphasis shifted from live vaccines to subunit vaccines whose duration of efficacy is time limited. Killed vaccines necessitate periodic re-vaccination.

Saying no to Pfizer was not as easy as it should have been.

When it comes to Crohn's disease, to its everlasting credit, the pharmaceutical industry identified the key factors in the inflammatory immune response and developed compounds that effectively blocked the target cytokine from effecting its objectives. These drugs have become collectively classified as biologics. In the treatment of chronic diseases for which they are used, they plicate, but do not cure!

AUTOIMMUNITY POSTULATE FOR CAUSATION

What trial and error attempts at therapy for Crohn's disease had documented was that causing impediment of the immune system's pro-inflammatory response resulted in an abatement of symptomology and evidence of mucosal healing. Using the resources at its command, the pharmaceutical industry dissected out the individual components of a pro-inflammatory response and constructed counter therapy to neutralize its net effect. This growing array of these compounds became collectively termed biologics. **The ability of biologics, steroids, and immunomodulators to induce temporary remissions is the foundational evidence for the autoimmune postulate of causation for Crohn's disease.**

- Suddenly, multiple journals whose titles included the word, autoimmunity, began publication. Without valid scientific substantiation, the label of autoimmunity was suddenly affixed to over a hundred disease entities. Crohn's disease became the poster-boy of autoimmunity. The application of that label circumvented the creative quest for causation. All the medical community needed to know was that a disease was due to autoimmunity. To make certain that was clearly understood, concerted effects were seemingly made to capture leadership.
- The assertion that Crohn's disease was mediated by an ongoing immune-mediated process is valid. The claim for causation is not. An immune mechanism of action requires not only an antibody/cytokine-mediated immune response, but a corresponding target antigen. The only candidate proposed was the gastrointestinal mucosa. This proposal was almost immediately discredited by the pathology of Crohn's disease. The initial gastrointestinal tissue damage is tightly focused in the ileocecal region. If the gastrointestinal mucosa was the target antigen, disease would occur throughout the small bowel. **What should have been the death blow to the autoimmunity paradigm was its nearly total inability to address the key WHYs embedded in the natural history of Crohn's disease.**

- Why the sudden appearance of a new disease?
- Why its epidemic spread globally?
- Why does breastfeeding provide protection against the future development of Crohn's disease?
- Why is disease initially limited to the ileocecal region?
- Why the absence of Crohn's disease in third-world economies until the introduction of western diet?

Without scientific confirmation, the pharmaceutical industry and its surrogates tenaciously advanced autoimmunity as their explanation for product use. The trials and tribulations of therapy with biologics dominate the gastrointestinal literature. In nearly two decades of utilization, biologics have not produced cures.

THE HRUSKA POSTULATE

USDA's reluctance to address the growing body of evidence for causality and the need to change the prevailing herd management schema prompted IDI to go outside of the United States to seek collaboration. IDI joined with the Veterinary Research Institute to pursue the issue of MAP and Crohn's disease.

The Veterinary Research Institute at Brno in the Czech Republic had been the intellectual powerhouse within the world of veterinary medicine. VRI's infectious disease section was led by an internationally acknowledged leader, Professor Karel Hruska. Using the institute's Centaur Global Network Information. Professor Karel Hruska monthly compiled and disseminated comprehensive lists of recent publication abstracts dealing with veterinary infectious diseases. In 2005, they identified that 49% of 51 brands of infant formula manufactured by 10 different producers in seven different countries contained MAP DNA. The paper's title read *"Mycobacterium avium* subsp. *paratuberculosis* in powdered infant milk: *paratuberculosis* in cattle—the public health crisis to be solved."* Their findings were re-corroborated by other investigators

The continued inability to get governmental regulatory agencies to address what had become an embarrassingly large body of work, prompted the mutual decision to weaponize VRI's Centaur Global Information Network (CGIN) in an attempt to break the dome of silence that governed dissemination of information dealing with MAP and Crohn's disease. CGIN disseminated IDI's 2012 White Paper of MAP and Crohn's disease as well as other unpublished data. On September 23, 2012, CGIN issued a call for mini-reviews on mycobacteria and Crohn's disease. In December of 2012, just prior to the release on VRI's Biomedical Technology, Epidemiology and Food Safety Network release of IDI's rebuttal to the pending OIE decision to remove MAP from the Terrestrial Animal Health Code and a companion letter from the president of the International Association for Paratuberculosis, the section's deputy directors and heads of the section were suddenly suspended without any reason being given.

Publication of CGIN ceased. In describing what happened, Professor Hruska wrote *"Details are not needed; nobody would believe them. It is a cruel life story like an absurd theatre."*

In 2014, Professor Hruska "accepted" retirement, but not before publishing, with Ivo, a paper entitled *"**Crohn's disease and related inflammatory diseases, from a single hypothesis to one "super hypotheses**."* If read in depth, this publication takes the mechanism that creates Crohn's disease into another realm. Professor Ivo Pavlik left the Institute.

Previously, one by one, the investigators that challenged the prevailing dogma had been silenced. Federal grants were cut or a University President had a private conversation with someone. With industry's iron hand now out of the glove, the option of slowly releasing scientific data pertaining to the causation of Crohn's disease was no longer an option. The **"VRI massacre" was a blatant bludgeoning of science that could not be allowed to quietly pass into the night**. Time constraints dictated that the entire story of Crohn's Disease be told now. The knowledge as to the specific elements that combined to produce Crohn's disease was rapidly published by IDI.

The pharmaceutical industry had rigged the system. It had gotten the FDA to agree that any administrative action/decision would be **evidence-based**. The translation of evidence based was a placebo-controlled, double blinded comparative study which achieved statistical significance whose cost runs into the millions of dollars. Only entities with that kind of fiscal fire-power could influence the topic.

History has documented that he who creates the experimental design can influence the outcome. The only counter to governance by designed experimentation was to document the Hruska postulate using experiments in nature whose validity could not be challenged. All the pieces to unraveling the causation of Crohn's disease and its transformation into a global epidemic were known. The infectious disease postulate of causation had identified the key player. The autoimmune postulates documented the presence of a dysfunctional proinflammatory response. Alone neither held water. Together they both gained traction. What had to be answered were:

Why did MAP have to become widespread among milking herds for Crohn's disease to occur?

Why was disease initially limited to the ileocecum and ascending colon?

Why the predilection for progressively younger and younger victims?

Intimate knowledge of congenital viral infection had demonstrated the absence of acquired immunity would transform a non-pathogen into a formidable disease entity.

Taking the mosaic of documented facts, the Hruska Postulate was constructed. The genesis of Crohn's disease begins when a newborn experiences significant MAP infectious challenge at a time when its acquired immunity has yet to develop. In order to abort continued MAP replication, the baby's genetically determined inherent immunity can become so stressed that its pro-inflammatory TH1 response against MAP becomes fixed within its immunological memory. That means that every time its immune system is presented with MAP, rather than responding with primarily a nonaggressive TH2 response (known as immunological tolerance), it again initiates a pro-inflammatory release of cytokines that attack MAP. In humans, MAP, unlike *Mycobacterium tuberculosis*, is a weak pathogen. The infectious inoculum must be sufficient that it stresses the baby's inherent immune system. Not every baby infected with MAP goes on to eventually develop Crohn's disease. The outcome is determined by inoculum size and genetically determined inherent immunity. Neonatal MAP infection transforms itself into a dysfunctional persistence of the proinflammatory response to Map. For disease to occur, the MAP antigen must be present. Hence the reason MAP must become widespread in the food supply to attain disease status.

While MAP receptor sites line the entire small bowel, MAP attachment is greatest in the region of maximum fecal stasis, the ileocecum. The pro-inflammatory immune response attacks MAP at its mucosal sites of attachment and antigen processing. The immense regenerative capacity reduces the resultant mucous damage to near insignificance; however, over time, if MAPs challenges are dense and frequent, the process eventually overwhelms the gastrointestinal tracts regenerative capacity and mucosal integrity is lost. This latter requisite stands to explain the long interim between creation of a dysfunctional pro-inflammatory response and the appearance of signs and symptoms of Crohn's disease.

More simply stated, **the absence of functional acquired immunity gives MAP infection the potential to convert itself from an infectious disease into an immune-mediated disease.**

The loss of mucosal integrity gives the gastrointestinal tract microbial flora an open portal for invasion. If left undertreated or untreated, the resultant polymicrobial bacterial invasion follows the principles of the anaerobic progression in which the many initial bacterial participants self-condense down to a few and within abscess to one organism. Continued bacterial replication creates the second pathological mechanism of disease production within Crohn's disease.

The early dominant bacteria are facultative anaerobes whose earmark is healing by fibrosis resulting in stricture and impaired small bowel motility. As the anaerobic progression shifts to the more obligatory anaerobes trans muscularis penetration allows segments of small bowel to adhere to each other and eventually become loop-to-loop fistula necessitating surgical intervention. Bowel rupture into the cul-de-sac can create perineal fistula. In the rush to deal with "inflammation" with just steroids or biologics, physicians often left the door open for the permanent sequela of Crohn's disease to develop

Why is Crohn' s disease a newly recognized disease entity: the progressive spread of MAP in dairy herds

Why does breastfeeding confer relative protection : reduced possibility of newborn MAP infection.

Why Crohn's disease is rare in third-world economies until the introduction of western diet: breastfeeding

Why the initial site of disease: increased mucosal attachment in the area of maximum small bowel stasis.

Why the global epidemic of Crohn's disease: the abandonment of breastfeeding and substitution of potentially MAP adulterated infant formula.

Why can't MAP be cultured or identified with special stains in diseased tissues containing MAP DNA: MAP resides a spheroclast (a bacteria without cell wall).

Why is Crohn's disease affecting children at progressively younger ages: increased density of MAP in the nation's food-supply.

Why can MAP be sometimes identified in the blood of a healthy individual: the person is in the active phase of a subclinical infection.

Why can MAP be occasionally demonstrated in normal small bowel: receptors for MAP line the entire small bowel given the widespread presence of MAP in the food supply, attachment will occur.

GASTROENTEROLOGY

The compartmentalization of medicine is such that the entry point for care of Crohn's disease is through gastroenterology. In theory, it is the depositor of clinical medical knowledge which is dispensed through the American College of Gastroenterology.

My initial orientation to gastroenterology was overwhelmingly positive. Frans Joseph Ingelfiner was Professor of Medicine at Boston University School of Medicine. Intellectually and physically he was a giant in his field. He would later become the editor of the New England Journal of Medicine. In my fourth year of medical school, I asked him to allow me to just follow him around as a fourth-year elective. After having given me a copy of a case presentation that he was about to give at the Boston City hospital, he asked me "What is the diagnosis". I CYA'd my answer, listing a number of possible explanations. Stopping in the middle of the street in front of the Boston City Hospital. He said "No". What is the diagnosis and Why?" Today, artificial intelligence does a better job than I did that day. But the medical bottom line has not. Circumstances within medical education have transformed the buildings of giants into that of Lilliputians.

From the 1960s to date, the inundation of information has resulted in a compartmentalization of medical knowledge. What that has created are islands of excellence surrounded by a sea of ignorance. Ask a cardiologist about a problem below the diaphragm or the next organ system over in the chest to discover major knowledge deficits. Specialists in internal medicine have become more body mechanics (BMs) than physicians.

The American College of Gastroenterology has taken the need to not understand big picture and internalized it. For nearly four decades, gastroenterologists have been the custodians of "inflammatory bowel diseases" for which they have no definite test and an equal amount of knowledge about the events that combined to create these diseases. Even more damning is their collective inability to effect cures. What they do know is how to treat inflammation: biologics and steroids. Today, inflammatory bowel disease (Crohn's disease and ulcerative colitis) constitutes a significant portion of gastroenterologists' income. Fortunately, collective ignorance has yet to be reflected in the discipline's fiscal standing: second only to cardiologists.

History has also been a poor teacher. Their prior experience with peptic ulcer disease should have engrained in their collective memory the knowledge that when you punch a hole through the gut, the gastrointestinal bacteria flora will make the patient pay dearly. Deaths associated with peptic ulcer disease were due to bleeding and Gram-negative sepsis.

When gastroenterologists treat Crohn's disease with biologics or steroids, and without any or with incomplete spectrum antibiotic coverage, they are relying on the 80% of the body's immunity and ultimate mucosal healing to take care of bacterial superinfection. Statistics tell us that 25% of afflicted individuals will have one or more operations in their lifetimes to remove diseased bowel. The immune-mediated process that causes local loss of mucosal integrity does not cause strictures, bowel obstruction, loop-to-loop anastomoses or perineal fistulae. Unless prior surgery has altered the placement of the small bowel, Ileocecal penetration results in the spillage of constituents of the gastrointestinal microbial flora into the cul-de-sac rather than the peritoneal cavity. **Strictures, loop-to-loop fistulae, perineal fistula and septic death are not the direct consequences of immune-mediated disease.**

History has not been kind to gastroenterologists. For three decades, peptic ulcer disease was the centerpiece of clinical practice in gastroenterology: a chronic disease. Their clinical practice took a big hit, when peptic ulcer was demonstrated to be a bacterial disease and curable. Then came "inflammatory bowel" disease. The growing fear among some gastroenterologists is that history is about to repeat itself.

In the past, gastroenterologists were independent contractors whose business hospitals attempted to recruit and whose ultimate allegiance was to the patient. Today, most gastroenterologists are not free to practice medicine in keeping with their knowledge and conscience. Working for corporative entities, they are employees who best adhere to governing guidelines of the institution and the discipline's leadership embodied in the American College of Gynecology. In 2018, the American College of Gastroenterology issued its Clinical Guideline (singular) for Crohn's Disease . It states *"Despite the recent advances in the treatment of patients with CD, there still remains a large group of patients who do not respond adequately to our current medication armamentarium."*............ *We will certainly expand our medical treatment war chest and uncover effective biologics with different mechanisms of action to treat our patient. If the initial biologic drug fails, the patient will be able to be switched to another agent and even combination biologics may become a reality."* The guideline further states that ***"the standard of care is rigid" and rarely violated"***.

A possible interpretation of this document could be viewed as stating that the standard-of-care is biologics forever and deviation from this guideline will render you legally vulnerable if something goes wrong.

THE PREVENTION OF CROHN'S DISEASE

The prevention of Crohn's disease is ridiculously simple, yet nearly impossible to achieve. The reasons have little to do with science.

The protective effect of breastfeeding for Crohn's disease has long been in evidence. Virtually, every retrospective study assessing risk factors for the development of Crohn's documented that breastfeeding confers a protective effect against the future development of Crohn's disease. When confronted with evidence of the role of infant formula in the apparent induction of a dysfunctional immune response, in its defense, Mead Johnson produced only one publication which did not demonstrate a protective effect. The study analyzed only Crohn's disease in older adults.

Retrospective epidemiologic studies are subjected to potential manipulative bias. Experiments in nature are not. The Canadian Indians, Maoris in New Zealand, Arab residents in Israel, the Gypsy populations and third-world nations, before the introduction of western food, all demonstrated the protection conferred by breastfeeding.

World War II and then the Iron Curtain, had isolated the Czech Republic from the world. Prior to 1950, MAP infection and paratuberculosis were virtually unknown in milking herds within the Czech Republic. Economic hardships forced most mothers to breastfeed their babies. Following the crumbling of the Iron Curtain, some 30,000 heifers were imported from countries whose herds contained animals with paratuberculosis. As the local economy improved, women began abandoning breastfeeding in favor of milk or infant formula. Initially, infant formula was produced from local herds; however, the single local producer was bought by an international company and local production was stopped. The domestic product was replaced by imported formula. In 2005, Hruska demonstrated that 49% of 51 brands of baby formula manufactured by 10 different producers in seven different countries contained the DNA of MAP. Between 1995 and 2004, the incidence of Crohn's disease in the Czech Republic increased 4.5-fold among 19+ year old and 6.5-fold in 65+ year old individuals.

Within the Czech Republic data, there existed an important embedded, control subpopulation: Roma (gypsies). Breastfeeding is culturally based among Roma women. Unlike their Czech counterparts, Roma women were much slower to adopt change. The rate of Crohn's disease among Roma has persistently been half the incidence of the rest of the Czech population.

In 2008, the **American Academy of Microbiologists** concluded that *"the association of MAP and CD (Crohn's disease) is no longer in question. The critical issue today is not whether MAP is associated with CD, but whether MAP causes CD or is only incidentally present".* Once the potential adulteration of infant formula by MAP had been documented and its significance became evidence-based, the manufacturers should have been under obligation to institute measures consistent with the precautionary principles regarding food safety embedded in The Rio Declaration and Article 5.7 of The World Trade Organization Agreement on Sanitary and Phytosanitary Measures. The manufacturers of infant formula had the options of 1) making certain that the milk powder used for their infant formula was MAP-free 2) develop a non-milk-based formula to be used for the first few weeks of a baby's life or 3) advocate that women not initially breastfeed their infants for the first four weeks of life.

Liability arising from the potential MAP contamination of milk and milk-based products will ultimately reside with the United States government. USDA's actions to insulate agribusiness from added costs by not identifying MAP status in an animal's health certificate allowed infected animals to be shipped across state and national borders. The USDA compounded the problem by licensing diagnostic tests that, at best, identified animals at risk for Johne's disease rather than being a statement as to whether or not the animal had been infected by MAP and the status of that infection. The net result has been the widespread dissemination of MAP among milk producing animals and the secondary shedding of MAP into the bulk tank milk.

Once the American Academy of Microbiologists declared that a relationship existed between MAP and Crohn's disease, USDA should have surrendered stewardship of the 2001 congressional mandate to either the National Institutes of Health or the Centers for Disease Control and Prevention.

The question of whether MAP in milk constitutes a public health hazard inadvertently resolved itself. The probability of an individual having been or being infected by MAP is but a function of diet and time. That the number of MAP infected individuals is only 1.2 million is consistent with the postulate that, **for individuals with intact immunity, MAP is a non-pathogen**. Pathogenicity expresses itself in individuals with acquired or congenital immunological deficiencies and newborns with incomplete acquired immunity.

In matters concerning food safety, The Rio Declaration on Food Safety and the World Trade Organization Agreement's Precautionary Principle had placed the obligation to protect the public welfare squarely on the FDA. Given that continued employment constitutes a desired objective, the presence of a viable, documented bovine pathogen in the nation's food supply created a dilemma for FDA. The agency buttressed itself against having to label a food substance as being hazardous or potentially hazardous to the public health by requiring that the **proof be first, evidence-based** and second, that the **proof be absolute**. Evidence-based usually translates as a double blind, placebo controlled, randomized comparative study with a statistically significant number of observations. Rigid adherence to this standard has allowed industry to control the preponderance of evidence-based knowledge. The other requisite, proof having to be absolute, has allowed a single contrarian publication to validate FDA's non-action in a given matter.

Tobacco being the primary cause of lung cancer is accepted as a "medical truth". Tobacco products come with a label stating that tobacco is hazardous to your health. That statement is not based upon absolute, non-contested proof or double blind, randomized comparative studies, but became actionable when the insurance companies made clear that the costs embedded in lung cancer therapy, litigation, and societal consequences exceeded tobacco's direct and indirect contributions to the national economy. Healthcare warnings against tobacco are based on scientific standards that have not been extended to MAP and Crohn's disease.

Teddy Roosevelt once said *"When a decision is required, the best thing to do is the right thing. The next best thing is to do the wrong thing. The worst decision is to do nothing".* With the passage of time and the progressive accumulation of pertinent data and the lack of contradicting data, the failure to do something about the Crohn's disease epidemic and its societal costs paints the leadership of the FDA in something less than a flattering light. Understanding the events that combine to produce Crohn's disease and the "medical truth" that breastfeeding confers relative protection against the future development of Crohn's disease would seemingly have **created an ethical imperative that a pregnant women be given the information that allows her to make a fully informed decision as to how her newborn will receive milk-based nutrition within the first four weeks of life**.

The Federal Meat Inspection Act (21 U.S.C. 601 et seq.), **the Poultry Protection Inspection Act** (21m U.S.C. 451 et seq.) and the Federal Food, Drug, and Cosmetic Act (21 U.S.C 321 et seq.) are instruments of administrative law. They identify a food as being adulterated if it bears or contains any poisonous or deleterious substance which may render it injurious to health and is not neutralized by its subsequent processing. Products that are adulterated under these laws cannot enter into commerce for food consumption.

Given the economic importance of milk derived protein and the adverse economic fallout from attempting to remove MAP adulterated food sources, made the U. S. government's decisions to not act understandable, but not allowing individuals the information necessary to make an informed decision became just one more instance in which **the public health has been subordinated to economics**. Even with IDI putting forth evidence of why MAP was a non-pathogen for individuals with intact immunity and that the Crohn's disease epidemic could be crippled by simply vigorously endorsing breastfeeding and providing the information necessary for a mother to make an informed decision as to whether or not to use infant formula, FDA's decision-making-process remained mute. Abraham Lincoln is once quoted to have said is *"To sin by silence when men (and women) should cry out makes cowards of men".* Viewed in the light of its societal consequences for human beings, FDA's silence on whether MAP constitutes a potential or real public health hazard soils its standing within the Public Trust.

Overall governmental disregard of its obligations within the Public Trust was in evidence in July of 2018. The U.S. delegation to the **United Nations-Affiliated World Health Assembly** stunned World Health officials by their "vigorous" opposition to the pending breastfeeding resolution. Decades of research had documented the superior health benefits of breastmilk over other products. A resolution to encourage breastfeeding was expected to have quick approval by the hundreds of government delegates gathered at the World Health Assembly. According to the article authored by Andrew Jacobs and published in the New York Times, the U.S. delegation upended the deliberations, demanding the removal of language that called on governments to protect, promote and support breastfeeding and to restrict the promotion of food products that may have deleterious effects on young children. The U.S. delegates defended their position by pointing out that not all women are able to breastfeed and by using formula, they could be stigmatized. When they failed, the delegation is said to have resorted to threats of punishing trade measures or withdrawal of military aid. Some delegates allegedly hinted that the United States threatened to cut its contribution to the World Health Organization. Ecuador, which had planned to introduce the measure, withdrew from doing so. When no other country volunteered to introduce the measure, Russia stepped in and introduced the resolution that the United States vigorously opposed. The resolution passed but not before the U.S. delegates had successfully removed language that called on the World Health Organization to provide technical support to member states seeking to halt inappropriate promotion of infant formula and had required the catch phrase **"evidence-based"** to be required for initiatives that promote breastfeeding. Restricting conclusions to **"evidence-based"** studies places the development of new ideas in the hands of those who fund **"evidence-based"** studies.

The lack of access to clean water that is mixed with powdered infant formula is estimated to indirectly be responsible for 800,000 infant deaths annually.

After the meeting, a policy director of the British advocacy group Baby Milk Action is quoted as having said *"We were astonished, appalled, and also saddened. ….."What happened was tantamount to blackmail, with the United States holding the world hostage and trying to overturn nearly 40 years of consensus on the best way to protect infant and young child health"*. What makes this ugly story uglier is that the U.S. delegates reputedly had access to the knowledge of infant formula's potential adulteration by MAP and of MAP's apparent causal relationship to Crohn's disease.

The **American Academy of Pediatrics and the Academy of Family Practice strongly advocated for breastfeeding.**

Given the knowledge that milk and infant formula can be adulterated by a documented bovine mycobacterium and that the preponderance of evidence pointed to an association between MAP and human disease, **FDA has basically sinned by silence by NOT requiring that a warning label be placed on infant formula.** FDA's ability to issue industry a *deus ex machina* protective ruling does not completely trump standing law. Based upon the preponderance of evidence for the causation of Crohn's disease and the statutes that require that all ingredients that could have a bearing on a consumer's decision to buy the product be listed, the manufacturers of infant formula were, and are, in apparent violation of marketing a defectively labeled product. Mothers are being denied the opportunity to make an informed decision as to whether or not they want their babies to be potentially exposed to MAP at a time when their immune system is incomplete has potentially serious legal ramifications.

Without a government upholding the precautionary principle, there can be no assurance of safety in what you eat. Crohn's disease is a prime example of **governmental negligent entrustment** that borders on being criminal.

Why intelligent leaders of federal agencies have become such invertebrates appears to be linked to *"The business of America is business"* and the political intervention by third-parties who apparently hold the federal agencies' prairie oysters in the palm of their collective hands.

THE CURING OF CROHN'S DISEASE

Temporary remission of disease is one thing. Permanent cure is another.

Steroids don't cure Crohn's disease. Biologics don't cure Crohn's disease. Isolated permanent remissions have occurred in individuals using dietary manipulation or having received anti-tuberculosis therapy.

In science, there is a rule that states that exceptions rewrite the governing rule.

We rarely read or cite the Japanese literature. In Japan, dietary manipulation had been an integral party of the primary therapy for Crohn's disease. Before the entrenchment of biologics as the standard-of-care, a few individuals afflicted with Crohn's disease had achieved permanent remission by rigid adherence to variations of basically vegetarian-like diets. In clinical trials of dietary manipulation, Chiba et al. reported that 94% of Crohn's afflicted individuals who remained on a semi-vegetarian diet maintained their clinical remission whereas 33% who returned to a regular diet relapsed. Sigall-Bonehet et al. reported that 70% of individuals with Crohn's disease achieved clinical remissions using exclusion diets. The Seattle group of pediatric gastroenterologists demonstrated a beneficial effect, but not cures through dietary manipulation. That diet is not an integral part of Crohn's disease therapeutics is due to the posturing of the American College of Gastroenterologists. The American College of Gastroenterology's 2018 Clinical Guide Line for Crohn's Disease omitted from reference and meaningful discussion the role of dietary manipulation.

What had not been in evidence was how the various dietary manipulations could act to alter disease manifestations in Crohn's disease. Then came the Hruska Postulate. The Hruska Postulate identified Crohn's disease as being a zoonotic food-borne disease due to *Mycobacterium avium* subspecies *paratuberculosis* (MAP). In the absence of functional acquired immunity, a newborn infected could be so challenged to abort mycobacterium replication that its inherent immune system became fixed within immunological memory. Owing to the loss of immunological tolerance, every time the baby's immune system encountered MAP, it would again respond by elaborating pro-inflammatory cytokines directed at MAP at its points of mucosal attachment to the gastrointestinal mucosa and its antigen processing. Much of the clinical response achieved by dietary exclusion of foods that had the potential of having been adulterated by MAP is due to reduction of mucosal antigen challenges.

An experiment-in-nature involving cow number 6140 which had far advanced terminal Johne's disease was destined to render an answer. In an attempt to prolong her life in order to collect added sera, she was put on an aggressive dietary supplementation that specifically targeted cellular immunity. Rather than dying in the anticipated two-three weeks, the animal staged more than a complete recovery. She thrived! Four months later her necropsy documented complete restoration of gastrointestinal structure. Not a single acid-fast bacilli characteristic of a mycobacterium was identified by two pathologists who examined some 24 slides. The massive infiltration of the lamina propria by eosinophils documented the mechanism by which the body can ultimately eliminate a mycobacterium. What had been done was remove stress and pushed a diet that enhanced her immune status.

In Crohn's disease, the diarrhea and loss of absorption areas cause significant loss of key vitamins and minerals vital to the integrity of host immunity. When analyzed individually, the exceptions that now define the rule had achieved their permanent clinical remissions through dietary manipulation that reverse a catabolic status and enhance host immunity.

In rare instances, permanent remissions have also been achieved using selected antimicrobials. The logical question becomes WHY?

The best endorsement that any proposed MAP therapeutic regimen could ask for is having the American College of Gastroenterology come out and specifically tell its members **not to use it**. Criticism can be flattery in disguise. In its 2018 Guideline for Crohn's disease, The American College of Gastroenterology' recommendation 15 reads:

"Anti-mycobacterial therapy has not been effective for induction or maintenance of remissions or mucosal healing in patients with Crohn's disease and **should not be used"**. ACG's *"extensive review of the published literature"* resulting in 375 references excluded key articles dealing with anti-MAP drug efficacy and nutritional therapy, passing undetected or not commented on. Medical publications with attention grabbing titles such as *"Anti-mycobacterium therapy in Crohn's disease: the end of a long controversy"* or *"Primary treatment of Crohn's disease: combined antibiotics taking center stage"* from respected investigators should have warranted either commentary or citation.

An Australian gastroenterologist, Thomas Borody, had apparently gotten under somebody's fiscal skin. Thomas Borody, is a medical Trekkie who is a gastroenterologist.. He thinks way outside of the box of medical dogma. He pioneered the use of fecal enemas to restore colic bacterial flora in cases of enterotoxigenic *Clostridium difficle* and other forms of colitis. Being a strong patient advocate, he critically analyzed the literature and came away with the conviction that, if the right combination of antimicrobials were used, he could cure individuals with Crohn's disease. Trying various combinations of antimicrobials, he was able to achieve prolonged, sustained remissions without continued therapy in individual patients. By way of mouth, the message got out. If you had Crohn's disease and wanted to be cured, go to Sidney, Australia.

One robin doesn't make a medical spring. Neither does two or even a few dozen. Dr. Borody put into evidence that, using selected antimicrobials, sustained, and presumably permanent remissions could be attained. Using capitalism to fight capitalism, Brody joined with RedHill Biopharma to successfully use his designated antimicrobial cocktail in several small studies. RHB-104 produced both mucosal healing and remissions when used in the treatment of treatment-naïve Crohn's disease. A prior major problem in the evaluation of antimicrobial therapy was the inclusion of afflicted individuals with complications due to bacterial superinfection. The problem was in interpreting the WHY. Borody's reasoning had been that Crohn's disease is due to MAP functioning as an infectious agent. For FDA,

RHB-104 hit the same stone wall as did the infectious disease postulate of causation. MAP can't be cultured or demonstrated by special stains in disease tissue containing MAP DNA.

The question now became HOW could these two divergent approaches to Crohn's disease, dietary manipulation and antimicrobial administration, attain same end result. The answer came from a single cow. Having far advanced Johne's disease, she became an animal of interest owing to her very high titer of anti-MAP antibodies. Under normal circumstances, her death would be anticipated in two or three weeks at most. In an attempt to prolong her life, she was removed from the herd and placed on a diet that targeted cellular immunity. Enhancement of host immunity destroyed MAP.

Why some antimycobacterial drugs worked while others failed had to do with their mechanism of action. The Hruska Postulate identifies the MAP template as being the engine responsible for the dysfunctional ongoing cytokine response to MAP. The identification of MAP DNA in diseased and lymphoid tissues represented MAP in its spheroplastic form. Destruction of the MAP template equates with the destruction of bacterial spheroplasts. Destruction of bacterial spheroplasts requires that antimicrobial therapy target its ribosomes. RHB-104 anti-MAP cocktail contains one or more compounds whose primary mechanism of action impedes ribosomal function. In contrast to anti-tuberculosis drugs that affect cell-wall synthesis, the success of antimicrobials that impact on RNA to induce mucosal healing and more sustained remission is the final piece that validates the Hruska postulate.

Both enhanced cellular immunity and selected anti-MAP therapy achieve permanent cures by the same mechanism, destroying the MAP templates that drive the dysfunctional immune response against *Mycobacterium avium* subspecies *paratuberculosis*. The importance of involving specialist in nutrition as part of the Crohn's disease team can not in any way be understated. Nutrition, more probably than not, is the key to shortening the interim between loss of mucosal integrity and its restoration.

WHY CROHN'S DISEASE IS NOT A CURABLE DISEASE

In today's medical world, **four aces do not beat a 45.**

The current therapy with biologics persists as the standard-of-care owing to the ability of third parties to control the dialogue. USDA did nearly everything possible to protect agribusiness from adverse fallout secondary to adulteration of milk and milk products by a certified bovine pathogen. In so doing, it unintentionally fueled the mechanism that produced an epidemic of Crohn's disease in children and young adults.

Using political leverage, third parties established the internal ruling that for FDA to act on a matter of public welfare, its decision had to be evidence-based. That sounds logical until the definition of evidence-based is spelled out; placebo controlled, double blinded, comparative studies that attained statistical significance. The multi-million-dollar cost of such studies leaves control of the experimental design in control of the study's sponsors.

In the real world, USDA and FDA don't make the rules. At the height of the AIDS epidemic, the director of the CDC advocated the use of condoms. One month later he was fired. An individual that I knew personally was installed. His qualifications for the office were ideological rather that meritorious.

To its credit, the pharmaceutical industry pulled off an amazing marketing coup with the biologics that is second only to UpJohn's marketing campaign for clindamycin. The company had developed clindamycin, an antibiotic with excellent coverage for anaerobic bacteria. The problem was that the average physician knew little to nothing about anaerobic infections. When UpJohn's marketing campaign was through, clindamycin was one of the leading antibiotics used in certain types of infections and made UpJohn a very considerable amount of money.

With biologics, the pharmaceutical industry went UpJohn one better. They developed products to fit the diseases whose defining characteristic was inflammation and then confabulated the rationale for the chronicity of their utilization. The myth of autoimmunity materialized. Entire journals devoted to the subject suddenly appeared. The availability of massive funding to study autoimmune disease inundated internal medicine. Individual physicians quickly made their reputations by championing autoimmunity. In 2019, Humira grossed 19.4 billion dollars. In the United States, the annual TV advertising for all biologics is in the hundreds-of-million dollars.

Any outcry relative to the cost of biologics is muted by having the tax payers unknowingly absorb the cost. Health insurance subsidizes the cost of biologics for those who can afford the premiums. For those unable to meet the cost of prolonged symptom suppression, particularly with Crohn's disease permanent sequela, they are forced to go on disability. By so doing, payment for the disease is shifted to the federal government (taxpayers). The estimated annual 15-17 billion dollars of direct medical costs and the added 25% of indirect medical costs for Crohn's disease detract significant funding from other national healthcare priorities.

Whether any censorship concerning MAP as the cause of Crohn's disease has been in place in the United States is highly debatable. Nevertheless, any publication which even touched on the possibility of a relationship between MAP and Crohn's disease did so lightly and carried with it the stock phrase "No relationship has been established". Subscriptions to libraries and advertising from the pharmaceutical industry constituted the primary funding of medical journals. Only after open publishing became mainstream, did articles directly addressing the pathogenesis of Crohn's disease appeared in U.S. medical journals: the Hruska postulate, the myth of autoimmunity, the permanent sequela of Crohn's disease being physician error, or curing Crohn's disease by destroying the MAP template. These concepts have gone unchallenged in the medical literature. The only tangible changes have been the increased funding of advertisements for biologics and the introduction of other biologics as drugs-of-choice for Crohn's disease as disenchantment with Humira emerged. Per the American College of Gastroenterology; "*Despite the recent advances* in the treatment of patients with CD, there still remains a large group of patients who do not respond adequately to our current medication armamentarium."............ We will certainly expand our medical treatment war chest and uncover effective biologics with different mechanisms of action to treat our patient. If the initial biologic drug fails, the patient will be able to be switched to another agent and even combination biologics may become a reality."

Dollars are bullets that target individuals who will develop Crohn's disease. In that regard, a 45 will beat science until someone says enough exploitation is enough and make it stick. Until then, it appears to be biologics forever.

BEYOND CROHN'S DISEASE AND AUTOIMMUNITY

Autoimmunity has been a mind paralyzing label that blocked the WHYs embedded in many other diseases.

The importance of the Hruska Postulate should not be understated. The Hruska Postulate identifies how an antigen challenge, in the absence of acquired immunity, can cause a fixation of the body's Th 1 pro-inflammatory response against the eliciting antigen to become fixed within immunological memory. **Crohn's disease had long been the poster-boy for autoimmunity.** What if Humira's (adalimumab), Entyvio's (vedolizumab), or Stelara's (ustekinumab)'s ability to transiently suppress but not cure diseases, are a tell that identify other curable immune-mediated diseases. Are rheumatoid arthritis, psoriasis, Hashimoto's thyroiditis, etc., etc., etc., etc. , immune-mediated diseases like Crohn's disease that are awaiting emancipation from investigative stagnation imposed by the label of autoimmunity?

YOU
CAN STOP CROHN'S DISEASE

If YOU don't have Crohn's Disease
    You can stop Crohn's disease by
        · Telling pregnant women to breast-fed their newborns for the first three to four weeks of life

If YOU have Crohn's Disease
        · Remove milk-based products and all meats that come that come from grass-fed animals from your diet *(dietary exclusion)*

        · Take daily vitamins C & D as well as biweekly zinc and selenium *(immune system enhancement)*

        · Add to your diet foods that enhance your body's immune system

        · Transfer your care to an internist with specialized training in infectious diseases. He or she is best qualified to treat submucosal bacterial infection and administer antimicrobial that appear to be effective in destroying the immune templates that drive the dysfunctional immune response *(physicians focused on curing disease)*

***" Insanity is to keep doing the same thing
and expecting a different result"***

KEY REFERENCES

Protective Effect of Breastfeeding

Bergstrand O., Hellers G. (1983). Breastfeeding during infancy in patients who later develop Crohn's disease. Scand. J. Gastroenterol, 18:903-906

Congilosi S. M., Rosendale D. E., Herman D. L. (1992) Crohn's disease – A rare disorder in American-Indians. West. J. Med. 157:682-683

Odes H. S., Locker C.,Neumann L., Zirkin H. J. et al. (1994) Epidemiology of Crohn's-disease in Southern Israel. M. J. Gastroenterol. 89:1859-1862

Corrao G., Tragnine A. Caprilli R. et al. (1998) Risk of inflammatory bowel disease attributable to smoking, oral contraception and breastfeeding in Italy: a nationwide case-control study. Intern. J. Epidemiol. 27:397-404

Niv Y. Abuksis G., Fraser G. M. (1999) Epidemiology of Crohn's disease in Israel; A survey of Israeli kibbutz settlements. Am. J. Gastroenterol. 94:2961-2965

Klement E., Cohen R. V., Boxman J. Joseph A. et al. (2004). Breastfeeding and risk of inflammatory bowel disease: a systemic review with meta-analysis. *Am J. Clin. Nutr.* 80:1342-1352

Hruska K., Pavlik I. (2004) Lower incidence of Crohn's disease in the Gipsy population of Hungary, the Maori population of New Zealand, Palestinians in Israel, Indians in Canada New Zealand. GME 2010, Kosice, Session 6 and Veterinarni Medicina

Thompson N. P., Montgomery S. M., Wadswoth, M. E. J. et al. (2005) Early determinants of inflammatory bowel disease: use of two national longitudinal birth cohorts, Eur. J. Gastroenteriol. Hepatol. 12:25-30

Karban A., Atia O., Leitersdorf E. et al. (2005) The relationship between NOD2/CARD 15 mutations and the prevalence and phenotypic heterogeneity of Crohn's disease: Lessons from Israeli Arab Crohn's Disease Cohort. Dig. Dis. Sci. 50:1692-1697

Ip S., Chung M., Raman G., Chew P. et al. (2007) Breastfeeding and maternal and infant health outcomes in developed countries, Evid. Rep. Technol. Assess. (Full Rep.) 153:1-186 ncbi.nlm.nih.gov/ Pubmed/17764214

Ip S., Chung M., Raman G., Chew P. et al. (2007) Breastfeeding and maternal and infant health outcomes in developed countries, Evid. Rep. Technol. Assess. (Full Rep.) 153:1-186 ncbi.nlm.nih.gov/ Pubmed/17764214

Barclay A. R., Russell R. K., Wilson M. L., et al. (2009). Systemic review: The role of breastfeeding in the development of pediatric inflammatory bowel disease. *J. Pediat.* 155:421-426.

Mikhailov T. A. (2009). Breastfeeding and genetic factors in the etiology of Crohn's disease. *World J. Gastroenterol.* 15:270-279.

Ponsonby A. L., Catto-Smith A. G., Pezic A. Dupuis S. et al. (2009). Association between early-I factors and risk of childhood onset of Crohn's disease among Victorian children born 1983-1998: a cohort study. *Inflam. Bowel Dis.* 15: 656-666

Hornell A., Lagstrom H., Lande B. Thorsdotti I.: (2013) Breastfeeding, introduction of other foods effect on health: a systemic review for the5th Nordic Nutrition Recommendations. Food Nut. Res. 57: 1-24

Horta B., Bahl R., Martinez J, Victora C. (2007). Evidence on the long-term effects of breastfeeding: systemic reviews and meta-analysis: World Health Organization: http://wholibdoc.who.int/publications/2007/9789241

Khalili H., Ananthakrishnan A. N., Higuchi L. M., et al. (2013) Early life factors and risk of inflammatory bowel disease in adulthood. Inflam. Bowel Dis. 19:542-547

Hornell A., Lagstrom H., Lande B., Thorsdottri I. (2013) Breastfeeding, introduction of other foods effect on health a systematic literature review for the 5th Nordic Nutrition Recommendations. Food Nut. Res. 5

Mycobacterium Avium subsp. Paratuberculosis

Schleig P. M., Buergelt C. D., Davis J. K., Williams E., Monif G. R. G., Davidson M. K.: 2005. Attachment of *Mycobacterium avium* subspecies *paratuberculosis* to bovine intestinal organ cultures: method of development of strain differences, Vet. Microbiol. 108:271-279

Eiichi M.2012. Epidemiological situation and control strategies for paratuberculosis in Japan. Japanese J. Vrt. Res. 60:19s-29s.

Monif G. R. G. 2008. Certification of health for dairy cows. ParaTb. Newsletter December p.3

Monif G. R. G. 2009. An ounce of prevention is worth more than a pound of cure: Certification of animals must be just that. ParaTb. December pp 40-41

Monif G. R. G., Williams J. E. 2015. Significance of single and double MAP agar gel immunodiffusion precipitation bands. Intern. J. Appl. Res. Vet. Med. 13:190-193.

Monif G. R. G., Williams J. E. 2013. The significance of a negative MAP ELISA test for Mycobacterium avium subspecies paratuberculosis. Intern. J. Appl. Vet. Res. 11:117-121

Monif G. R. G., Williams J. E. 2015. Relationship of intestinal eosinophilia and acid-fast bacilli in Johne's disease. Intern. J. Appl. Res. Vet. Med. 13: 147-148.

Mycobacterium Avium subsp. Paratuberculosis and Milk

Ahrens P. (2000) Detection of *Mycobacterium avium* subsp. *paratuberculosis* in milk from clinically affected cows by PC7R and culture. Vet. Microbiol. 77:291-297

Pinedo P. J., Williams J. E., Monif G. R. G. (2008) *Mycobacterium paratuberculosis* shedding into milk: association of ELISA seroreactivity with DNA detection in milk. Intern. J. Appl.Res. Vet. Med. 6:137-144

Ellingson J.L., Anderson J.L., Koziczkowski J.J. (2005) Detection of viable *Mycobacterium avium* subspecies *paratuberculosis* in retail pasteurized whole milk by two culture methods and PCR. J. Food Prot. 2005: 68:966-972.

Ayele W.Y., Svastova P, Roubal P., et al. (2005) *Mycobacterium avium* subspecies *paratuberculosis* cultured from locally and commercially pasteurized cow's milk in the Czech Republic. Appl. Envir. Microbiol. 2005; 71:1210-1214

Grant I. R., Ball H. J., Rowe M. T. (2002) Incidence of *Mycobacterium paratuberculosis* in bulk raw and commercially pasteurized milk from approved dairy processing establishments in the United Kingdom. Appl. Envir. Microbiol. 68:2428-2435

Clark D. L. Jr., Anderson J. L., Kozickowski J. J., Ellingson J. L. E. (2006) Detection of *Mycobacterium avium* subspecies *paratuberculosis* in cheese curds purchased in Wisconsin and Minnesota. Molecular Cell. Probes 20:197-202

Ikonomoplus J., Pavilk I., Bartos M. et al. (2005)Detection of *Mycobacterium avium* subspecies *paratuberculosis* in retail cheese from Greece and Czech Republic. Appl. Environ Microbiol. 71:8935-9036

Hruska K., Baros M., Kralik P., Pavlik I. (2005) *Mycobacterium avium* subspecies *paratuberculosis* in powdered infant milk: paratuberculosis in cattle – the public health problem to be solved. Veterinarni Medicina 50:327-335-230

Donaghy J.A., Johnston J., Rowe M. T. 2011 Detection of *Mycobacterium avium* ssp. *paratuberculosis* in cheese, milk powder, and milk using IS900 and f57-based qPCR assays. J. Appl. Microbiol. 110:479-489

Millar, D. Ford, J. Sanderson, J. et al. 1996. IS 900 PCR to detect *Mycobacterium avium* subspecies *paratuberculosis* in retail supplies of whole pasteurized milk in England and Wales. Appl. Environ Microbiol. 62:3446-54

Monif, G. R. G. 2016. Hypothetical liability from MAP causing Crohn's disease. ParaTB Newsletter. pp 18-18.

The Story of Crohn's Disease

Chiodini Rossier C. A. 1996: Paratuberculosis: a potential zoonosis. Vet. Clin. North Am.: Food Animal Practices 12:457-467

Herman-Taylor J. 2000 Mycobacterium avium subspecies paratuberculosis in the causation of Crohn's disease World J. Gastroenterol; 6:630-63

Bull T. L., McMinn E. J., Sid-Boumedine K. et al. 2003. Detection and verification of *Mycobacterium avium* subspecies *paratuberculosis* in fresh ileocolonic mucosal biopsies from individuals with and without Crohn's disease. J. Clin. Microbiol; 41:2915-23.

Naser S. A., Schwartz D., Shafran I. 2000. Isolation of Mycobacterium avium subspecies paratuberculosis (MAP) from the breastmilk of patients with Crohn's disease. Amer. J. Gastroenterol. 95:1094-1095

Naser S. A., Ghobrial G., Romero C., Valentine F. 2004 Culture of *Mycobacterium avium* subsp. *paratuberculosis* (MAP) from the blood of Crohn's disease patients. Lancet 364: 1039-1044.

Scana A. M., Bull T. J., Cannas S., Sanderson J. D., Sechie LA, et al. *Mycobacterium avium* subspecies *paratuberculosis* infection of irritable bowel syndrome comparison with Crohn's disease: common neural and immune pathogeniciities. J. Clinical Microbiol. 2007: 45:3883-90

Sechi L. A., Scana A. M., Molicottie P. et al 2005. Detection and isolation of *Mycobacterium avium* subspecies *paratuberculosis* from intestinal biopsies of patients with and without Crohn's disease in Sardinia. Am. J. Gastroenterol. 100:1529-34.

Juste R. A., Elguezabal N., Pavon A . et al. 2009. Association of *Mycobacterium avium* subspecies *paratuberculosis* DNA in blood and cellular and humeral Immune response in inflammatory bowel disease patents and controls, Int. J. Infect. Dis. 13: 247-254.

Monif G. R. G. 2015 The Hruska postulate of Crohn's disease. Med. Hypothesis 85:878-881

Monif, G. R. G. 2016. The Mycobacterium avium subspecies paratuberculosis dilemma. Biol. Med. 8:2-5. Doi.org/10.4172097-8369 1000270

Monif, G. R. G. (2017) An infectious disease process within an immune-mediated disease process: The role of the gastointestinal microbiota in Crohn's disease. Adv. Res. Gastroenterol. Hepatology 5 (5) : ARGH NS555675

Monif G. R. G.: Translation of hypotheses to therapy in Crohn's disease. J. Inflam. Bowel Dis. & Disorder 2016; 1:1 doi.org//10.4172/JIBDD.10002

Monif G. R. G.: 2017. The prevention of Crohn's disease. Adv. Res. Gastroenterol. Hepatol. 8(3):-2 doi:10.19080/ARGH.2017.08.555738

Monif G. R. G. 2018. The quest for a cure to Crohn's disease. Adv. Med. Biol.129:187-204

Monif G. R. G. 2018. The myth of autoimmunity. Med. Hypothesis.121:78-79 doi.org/10.1016/.mehy.2018.09.023

Monif G. R. G., 2018. Understanding therapeutic concepts in Crohn's disease. Clin. Med. Insights Gastroenterol. 20:1-3. Doi.10.1177/1179552218815169

Monif G. R. G. 2018. Are the permanent sequelae of Crohn's disease a failure to treat the gastrointestinal microbiota. Med. Hypothesis. 122:198-199

Monif G. R. G. 2018. The paradigms of causation for Crohn's disease. J. Infect. Dis. Immune Ther. 1:1-3 open access

Monif, G. R. G. 2017. An infectious disease process within an immune-mediated disease process: The role of the gastointestinal microbiota in Crohn's disease. *Adv. Res. Gastroenterol. 2 Hepatology* 5 (5) :ARGH NS555675

Monif . R. G.2018. The WHY? Of Crohn's disease. Adv. Res. Gastroenterol. Hepatpol. 10 (5) doi.10.19080/Argh.2018 10.555798

Monif G. R. G. 2018 The theoretical antibiotic selection for the polymicrobial infection of Crohn's disease. Adv. Res. Gastroenterol. Hepatpol.. 10 (2) doi;10.19080/ARGH.2018.10.555785

Monif G. R. G. 2018 Undertreating polymicrobial infection in Crohn's disease. J. Trans. Gastroenterol. Clin. Hepatol. Doi. 10.31021/jtgch.20181106

Monif G. R. G. 2020. MAP template controlling Crohn's disease. Med. Hypothesis 138. doi.org/10.1016/j.mehy, 2020.109593

United States Department of Agriculture (USDA)

United States voluntary Johne's disease herd status program for cattle. 2000. United States Animal Health Association www.aphis.usda.org/njwg/jddairym.html

Uniform program standards for the voluntary Johne's disease control program. United States Department of Agriculture Animal and Plant Health Inspection Service. APIS 91-45-014

Stabel J. R., Steadham E. M. Bolin C. A. 1997. Heat inactivation of *Mycobacterium paratuberculosis* in raw milk: are current pasteurization conditions effective? Appl. Environ. Microbiol. 63:975-977

United States Department of Agriculture Animal Plant Health Inspection Service. 2000. 9 CFR Parts 71 and 80. Johne's disease in domestic animals; interstate movement. Federal Register 65:18875-18879

USDA-APHIS Johne's Disease in U.S. Dairies 1991-2007. http://nahms.aphis. usda.pov/dairv/dairvolfDairv 2007-Johnes.pdf.

Schwartz A. 2008. National Johne's Disease Control Program Strategic Plan. U.S/Animal Health Association. October 23, 2008 (http://www.johne'sdisease. org/2008.StrategicPlan.pdf)

Monif G. R. G. 2018. Retrospective Assessment of USDA Steward ship of Mycobacterium avium subspecies paratuberculosis dilemma. ParaTB. Newsletter. July 2018, pp 4-8

Dietary Manipulation and Crohn's Disease

Hruska K., Baros M., Kralik P., Pavlik I.: *Mycobacterium avium* subspecies *paratuberculosis* in powdered infant milk: paratuberculosis in cattle – the public health problem to be solved. Veterinarni Medicina 2005; 50:327-335-230

Suskind D. L. Wahbeh G. Cohen S. A. et al. 2016. Patients perceive clinical benefit with specific carbohydrate diet for inflammatory bowel disease. Dig. Dis. Sci. 61:3255-3260

Cohen S. a., Gold D. B., Oliva S. et. al 2014. Clinical and mucosal improvement with specific carbohydrate diet in pediatric Crohn's disease. J. Pediatr. Gastroenterol. 59:516-521

Burgis J. C., Nguten K., Park K. T., Cox K. 2016. Response to strict and liberalized specific carbohydrate diet in Pediatric Crohn's disease. World J. Gastroenterol. 22:211-2117

Penagin F., Dilillo D., Borsani B., et al. 2016. Nutrition in pediatric inflammatory bowel disease: From etiology to treatment. A systemic review. Nutrients 1:8. doi. 10.3390/nu8060334

Romano A., Castagna V. 2016. Human nutrition from the gastroenterologist's perspective. Gastroenterol. Clin. N. Amer. Page 79-86

Monif G. R. G., Williams J. E. 2015. Relationship of intestinal eosinophilia and acid-fast bacilli in Johne's disease. Intern. J. Appl. Res. Vet. Med. 13:147-149

Buergelt C. D., Williams J. E., Monif G.R. G. 2004. Spontaneous clinical remission of Johne's disease in a Holstein cow. Intern. J. Appl. Res. Vet. Med. 2:126-128

Monif G. R. G. 2017. The enhanced role of diet in Crohn's disease. Adv. Res. Gastroenterol. Hepatology. 3:ARGH NS55529

Valberg L. S., Flanagan P. R., Kertesz A., Bondy D. C. 1986. Zinc absorption in inflammatory bowel disease. Dig. Dis. Sci. 32:724-731

McClain C. J., Soutor C., Hiornig D. H. 1980. Zinc deficiency: a complication of Crohn's disease. Gastroenterol. 78:273-279

Girodon F., Galan P., Monget A. L. et al. 1999. Impact of trace elements and vitamin supplementation on immunity and infection in the elderly institutionalized patients: a randomized controlled trial. MIN VITAOX. Arch. Intern. Med. 159:748-754

Wintergerst E. S., Maggini S., Hiornig D. H. 2007. Contribution of selected vitamins and trace elements to immune function Ann. Nutri. Metab. 51: 301-323

Chiba M., Abe T., Tsuda H. et al.2010. Lifestyle-related diseases in Crohn's disease:relapse prevention with semi-vegetarian diet. Wor[d J. Gastroenterol. 16:2484-2495

Sigall-Bonch R., Pfeffer-Gik T., Segal I. 2014 .Parenteral enteric nutrition with Crohn's disease exclusion diet is effective for induction of remission in children and young adults.Infam. Bowel Dis. 20:1353-1360

Antimicrobial Therapy and Crohn's Disease

M. A., Hanley J. 2008. Anti-mycobacterial therapy for Crohn's disease: a reanalysis. Lancet Infect. Dis. 8:34

Chamberlin W., Borody T. J., Campbell J. 2011. Primar ytreatment of Crohn's disease: combine antibiotics taking center stage. Expert. Rev. Clin. Immunol. 7:761-759

Biroulet I. P., Neut C., Colombel J. F. 2008. Anti-mycobacterium therapy in Crohn's disease: the end of a long controversy? Prac. Gastroenterol. 1:11-17

Williams J. E., Monif G. R. G. 2008. Impact of immunonutritional dietary additives on AGID positive cows with Johne's disease. Paratub Newsletter March 7-8.

Warren J. E., Rees H., Cox T. 1986 Remission of Crohn's disease with tuberculosis therapy N. Engl. J. Med 214:182.

Borody T. J. , Bilkey S., Wettstein A. R., et al. 2007 Anti-mycobacterial therapy in Crohn's disease heals mucosa with longitudinal scars. Dig. Liver Dis. 39:438-444.

Chamberlin W., Ghobrial G., Chehtane M., et al. 2007. Successful treatment of a Ceohn's disease patient with bacterium paratuberculosis. Am. J. Gastroenterol 102-689-691.

Shafran I., Burgeunder P. 2008. Rifaximin for the treatment of newly diagnosed Crohn's disease: A case series. Am J Gastroenterol 103:2158-2160.

Lipton J. E. 2012. My personal MAP-quest. ParaTb.Newsletter June 17-18.

Agrawal G., Clancy A., Sharma R. 2020. Targeted combination antibiotic therapy induces remission in treatment-naïve Crohn's disease: A case series J.; Microorganisms 8:371 Doi.org/103390/microorganisms8030371

NTBR

Nancy C., Buckley M. 2008. Mycobacterium avium subspecies paratuberculosis: Infrequent Human Pathogen or Public Health Threat? Report from the American Academy of Microbiology 1-37

Botkin J. R. 2018 Should failure to disclose significant financial conflict of interest be considered research misconduct. JAMA 320:2307-2308. Doi:10:1001/jama.2018.17525

Cigarro F. G., Masters B.S., Sharphorn D. 2018 Institutional conflict of interest and the public trust. JAMA 329-2305-2306. Doi:10.1001/JAMA.2018.18412

Ornstein C. Thomas K. 2018. The New York Times. What these medical journals don't reveal: Top doctor's ties to industry, December 8. 2018

www.ingramcontent.com/pod-product-compliance
Lightning Source LLC
Chambersburg PA
CBHW060520280326
41933CB00014B/3045